Healing Herbs for Diabetes

Harnessing Nature's Remedies for Natural
Management and Reversal of Diabetes through
Cultivation and Utilization

J. Waller

J. Waller

© [2024] J. Waller. All rights reserved.

No part of this book may be reproduced, distributed, or transmitted in any form or by any means, including photocopying, recording, or other electronic or mechanical methods, without the prior written permission of the author, except in the case of brief quotations embodied in critical reviews and certain other noncommercial uses permitted by copyright law.

.

Healing Herbs for Diabetes

Introduction _____ *6*

    Overview of Diabetes: Definition, Types, and Prevalence ____ 6

    The Importance of Natural Remedies _____ 9

    Objectives of the Book _____ 11

Chapter One: Understanding Diabetes and Its Management _____ *15*

    Diabetes Pathophysiology: How Diabetes Affects Your Body 15

    The Role of Insulin _____ 15

    Complications of uncontrolled diabetes _____ 17

    Medications for Diabetes _____ 19

    The Role of Nutrition: Importance of Diet in Managing Diabetes _____ 23

    Integrating Herbs into Your Diet _____ 27

Chapter 2: Herbal Remedies for Diabetes _____ *29*

    Factors to Consider When Choosing Herbs for Diabetes ____ 29

    Overview of Effective Herbs: A Short Introduction to Key Herbs Used in Diabetes Management _____ 34

Chapter 3: Key Healing Herbs. _____ *41*

    Preparation Techniques and Dosage Recommendations ____ 42

Safety and interactions with other medications _____ 46

How To Consume and Apply Aloe Vera _____ 47

Traditional Applications and Modern Research Findings ___ 48

Active Ingredients and Benefits _____ 49

Culinary Uses and Supplements _____ 50

Chapter 4: Growing Healing Herbs. _____ *54*

Starting Your Herbal Garden _____ 54

Basic Gardening Tips for Beginners _____ 56

Chapter 5: Using Herbs in Daily Life. _____ *62*

Incorporating herbs into meals _____ 62

Herbal Tea and Supplements _____ 67

Creating herbal remedies _____ 71

Chapter 6: Lifestyle Changes for Diabetes Management. _ *77*

Integrating Herbal Remedies, Diet, and Exercise _____ 77

Mindfulness & Stress Management _____ 81

Practicing mindfulness _____ 82

Establishing a Monitoring Routine _____ 86

Communicate with Your Healthcare Team _____ 87

Healing Herbs for Diabetes

Chapter 7: Safety Considerations. _____ 89

Possible Side Effects of Herbs _____ 89

Interactions with medications _____ 93

Understanding Herbal-Drug Interactions _____ 93

Personalized Approaches _____ 96

Conclusion _____ 100

Empowerment via Knowledge _____ 100

Last Thoughts on Managing Diabetes Naturally _____ 102

The end _____ 106

Introduction

Overview of Diabetes: Definition, Types, and Prevalence

Diabetes mellitus, or simply diabetes, is a chronic medical illness characterized by elevated blood sugar (glucose) levels. This disorder develops when the body either generates insufficient insulin or is unable to adequately use the insulin it does produce. Insulin is a hormone generated by the pancreas that helps glucose move from the bloodstream to the body's cells, where it is used for energy. When this process is disturbed, it might result in major health consequences if not addressed properly.

Healing Herbs for Diabetes

There are three main forms of diabetes:

Type 1 diabetes is an autoimmune condition in which the immune system mistakenly assaults and destroys insulin-producing beta cells in the pancreas. It commonly develops in children and young adults, thus the old term "juvenile diabetes." Individuals with Type 1 diabetes require insulin therapy for the rest of their lives to survive.

Type 2 diabetes, the most prevalent kind of diabetes, develops when the body becomes insulin resistant or the pancreas fails to generate enough insulin. This type is frequently associated with lifestyle problems such as obesity, sedentary behavior, and poor food. It is most commonly diagnosed in adults, although rising obesity rates have resulted in an increase in instances among children and adolescents.

Gestational diabetes develops during pregnancy when the body's insulin production is insufficient to meet the increased demands of both the mother and the developing fetus. While gestational diabetes often cures after childbirth, it can raise the mother's chance of acquiring Type 2 diabetes later in life.

Diabetes has reached epidemic proportions globally. According to the International Diabetes Federation, roughly 537 million persons aged 20 to 79 had diabetes in 2021, with the total expected to climb to 783 million by 2045. Factors contributing to this substantial increase include urbanization, sedentary lifestyles, poor food choices, and rising obesity rates. Diabetes is more than just a personal health issue; it poses substantial difficulties to public health systems and economies around the world.

Healing Herbs for Diabetes

The Importance of Natural Remedies

Given these astonishing statistics, the search for improved diabetes control and potential reversal has received a great deal of interest. While traditional medicine has made significant progress in treating diabetes, including the development of insulin therapy and oral drugs, many people are looking for complementary and alternative treatments. This trend reflects an increasing knowledge of natural medicines' potential benefits, as well as a desire for holistic solutions.

Natural therapies, particularly herbal treatments, have been used for centuries in many civilizations around the world. Many herbs have qualities that can help regulate blood sugar levels, increase insulin sensitivity, and address other underlying causes of diabetes. According to research, many herbs, including bitter melon, cinnamon, and fenugreek, have active components that may have a good impact on glucose metabolism and overall health.

In recent years, there has been a resurgence of interest in herbal medicine, motivated by factors such as:

Growing distrust in pharmaceuticals: Concerns about side effects, reliance, and the expensive expense of medications have prompted people to look for alternative treatments.

Increased access to information: The internet and social media have made it easier for people to find and share information about herbal medicines.

Desire for holistic health: Many people want to improve their overall well-being by incorporating natural medicines into their routines as preventive measures.

Healing Herbs for Diabetes

The use of herbal remedies into diabetes management can provide various advantages, including fewer side effects, a higher quality of life, and a more individualized approach to healthcare. However, these therapies must be approached with caution because not all plants are suitable for everyone and can combine with conventional pharmaceuticals.

Objectives of the Book

This book, "Healing Herbs for Diabetes: Harnessing Nature's Remedies for Natural Management and Reversal of Diabetes through Cultivation and Utilization," seeks to provide a complete resource for anyone who want to harness the force of nature in their fight against diabetes. This book aims to provide readers with knowledge and skills to take control of their health by investigating the potential of various herbs, the cultivation methods required to grow these plants, and practical applications for their use.

This book's objectives are as follows:

Educating Readers About Diabetes: Providing a basic overview of diabetes, including its various forms, symptoms, complications, and traditional treatments, to assist readers comprehend the significance of management measures.

Exploring Healing Herbs: Learn about certain herbs that have been shown to be effective in diabetes management, including their active components, health benefits, preparation techniques, and recommended dosages. Each herb discussed in this book will be supported by scientific study and historical usage.

Cultivation Techniques: Provides practical guidance on how to grow healing herbs at home,

Healing Herbs for Diabetes

regardless of gardening experience. This section will help readers establish their own herbal gardens by covering everything from plant selection to soil requirements and care.

Practical applications include easy-to-follow recipes and strategies for incorporating herbs into everyday life. This includes instructions for making herbal teas, tinctures, and other medicines, as well as adding herbs into meals to maximize their health advantages.

Holistic Lifestyle adjustments: Readers are encouraged to take a complete approach to diabetes control that includes food adjustments, exercise, stress management, and herbal medicines.

Safety and Interactions: Educating readers on the significance of speaking with healthcare practitioners before introducing herbs into their diabetes treatment regimen, as well as highlighting potential adverse effects and interactions.

By the end of this book, readers will have the information and tools they need to make informed decisions about including herbal therapies into their diabetes control plans. Whether you are newly diagnosed, looking for alternative therapies, or looking to improve your current regimen, this book is intended to be a reliable companion on your journey to greater health.

Chapter One: Understanding Diabetes and Its Management

Diabetes Pathophysiology: How Diabetes Affects Your Body

Diabetes mellitus, sometimes known as diabetes, is a chronic disorder that affects how the body metabolizes glucose, a primary source of energy. Understanding the pathophysiology of diabetes is critical for understanding its health consequences and the importance of effective management strategies.

The Role of Insulin

The pancreas produces the hormone insulin, which is central to diabetes. Insulin regulates blood sugar levels by allowing glucose to enter cells and be used for energy. A healthy person's pancreas produces insulin in reaction to increased blood glucose levels, such as after eating. However, in people with diabetes, this process is interrupted.

Type 1 diabetes develops when the immune system attacks and destroys insulin-producing beta cells in the pancreas. As a result, the body generates little or no insulin, causing high blood glucose levels. This kind is frequently diagnosed in children and young adults, thus the prior term "juvenile diabetes."

Type 2 diabetes occurs when the body becomes insulin resistant or fails to produce enough insulin to maintain normal glucose levels. Obesity, physical inactivity, and heredity all have a role in the progression of Type 2 diabetes. This kind of

Healing Herbs for Diabetes

diabetes is frequently associated with lifestyle choices and is more common in adults, but rising incidence among children and adolescents are causing worry.

Complications of uncontrolled diabetes

Diabetes, if not treated properly, can cause major health consequences affecting many organs and systems throughout the body. High blood glucose levels can harm blood vessels, nerves, and tissues, resulting in:

Diabetes increases the risk of heart disease and stroke due to elevated triglyceride and LDL cholesterol levels.

Neuropathy: High blood sugar levels can damage nerves, especially in the extremities, causing pain, tingling, or loss of sensation.

Diabetic retinopathy is a condition in which high blood sugar levels damage the blood vessels in the retina, potentially causing blindness.

Diabetes can induce nephropathy, which decreases kidney function and eventually leads to renal failure.

Poor Wound Healing: High blood sugar levels can impair the body's capacity to heal wounds, raising the risk of infections and amputations, especially in the foot.

The combined effects of these issues highlight the important need for appropriate management measures to keep blood glucose levels within normal limits.

Conventional Treatments: A Review of Medications and Lifestyle Changes

Healing Herbs for Diabetes

Diabetes is normally managed with a mix of medications, lifestyle adjustments, and monitoring. Conventional treatments try to keep blood glucose levels within therapeutic limits, lowering the risk of complications and enhancing quality of life.

Medications for Diabetes

Insulin therapy is crucial for people with Type 1 diabetes to survive. Insulin can be provided via injections or insulin pumps, and there are several varieties available, including rapid-acting, short-acting, intermediate-acting, and long-acting insulin. Insulin regimens are adjusted to each individual's needs, lifestyle, and preferences.

For patients with Type 2 diabetes, a variety of oral drugs are available to assist regulate blood sugar levels. This includes:

Metformin, a first-line drug, enhances insulin sensitivity and lowers glucose synthesis by the liver. It is generally well tolerated and may aid with weight management.

Sulfonylureas: These drugs help the pancreas make more insulin. Examples are glipizide and glyburide.

DPP-4 Inhibitors: These drugs, such as sitagliptin, stimulate insulin synthesis while decreasing glucose release from the liver in response to meals.

GLP-1 Receptor Agonists: These injectable drugs, such as liraglutide, imitate the effects of the GLP-1 hormone, which stimulates insulin secretion and slows stomach emptying, promoting satiety and weight loss.

SGLT2 Inhibitors: This type of drug, which includes empagliflozin, acts by inhibiting glucose

Healing Herbs for Diabetes

reabsorption in the kidneys, resulting in increased glucose excretion in the urine.

It is crucial to remember that medication selection is extremely customized and should be discussed with a healthcare provider.

Lifestyle changes are the cornerstone of management.

In addition to medicine, lifestyle adjustments are essential for diabetes management. Key areas include:

Diet: Following a well-balanced diet rich in whole grains, lean proteins, healthy fats, fruits, and vegetables can have a substantial impact on blood sugar levels. It is critical to monitor carbohydrate intake since carbs have the greatest direct effect on blood glucose.

Physical Activity: Engaging in regular physical activity is critical for maintaining a healthy weight and increasing insulin sensitivity. The American Diabetes Association recommends at least 150 minutes of moderate-intensity aerobic exercise each week, including strength training at least twice a week.

Weight Management: Achieving and maintaining a healthy weight can help with blood sugar control and lower the risk of problems. Even modest weight loss (5-10% of body weight) can have a major impact on those with Type 2 diabetes.

Monitoring Blood Sugar Levels: Regular blood glucose monitoring allows people to understand how their bodies react to foods, drugs, and exercise. This information is critical for making sound decisions about lifestyle and treatment changes.

Stress Management: Chronic stress might lower blood sugar levels. Stress-reduction techniques such as mindfulness, meditation, or yoga can help people manage their diabetes more efficiently.

The Role of Nutrition: Importance of Diet in Managing Diabetes

Nutrition is extremely important in diabetes management. A well-balanced diet not only helps to control blood sugar levels, but it also promotes overall health and well-being. Understanding the link between food and diabetes is critical for making sound dietary decisions.

Essential Dietary Principles for Diabetes Management

Carbohydrate Counting: Because carbs have the greatest impact on blood glucose, understanding how to count carbohydrates is critical for those with diabetes. This includes being conscious of serving sizes and carbohydrate levels in foods. Food diaries and mobile applications can help you keep track of your intake.

Glycemic Index (GI): The glycemic index determines how rapidly carbohydrate-rich diets elevate blood sugar levels. Foods with a high GI are rapidly absorbed, resulting in increases in blood glucose, whereas low-GI foods cause a slower, more steady increase. Low-GI foods including whole grains, legumes, and non-starchy vegetables can help keep blood sugar stable.

Portion Control: Portion control is essential for avoiding excessive calorie intake and regulating weight. Using measuring cups, food scales, and mindful eating techniques can help with portion control.

Healing Herbs for Diabetes

A balanced meal includes a variety of carbohydrates, proteins, and healthy fats. Incorporating lean proteins (such as fish, chicken, and plant-based sources), healthy fats (such as nuts, seeds, and avocados), and a range of colorful fruits and vegetables can help you obtain more nutrients and feel better overall.

Hydration: Staying hydrated is vital for proper bodily function. Water should be the preferred beverage, with sugary drinks and caffeine consumption strictly regulated.

Mindful Eating: Paying attention to hunger indicators, appreciating flavors, and minimizing distractions can improve the eating experience and help people make healthier choices.

Superfoods and Diabetes Management

Certain foods are particularly healthy for those with diabetes, frequently referred to as "superfoods." These include:

Leafy Greens: Spinach, kale, and collard greens are low in calories and carbs, but high in important nutrients and fiber.

Berries: Strawberries, blueberries, and raspberries are high in antioxidants and have a lower glycemic index than other fruits, making them an ideal snack.

Nuts and Seeds: Almonds, walnuts, and chia seeds are high in healthy fats, protein, and fiber, which can help regulate blood sugar levels.

Whole grains, such as quinoa, barley, and brown rice, provide fiber and important minerals while lowering blood sugar levels when compared to refined grains.

Legumes: Beans, lentils, and chickpeas are high in protein and fiber, making them good choices for satiety and blood sugar control.

Integrating Herbs into Your Diet

As we investigate the efficacy of herbal medicines in the next chapters, it is critical to recognize herbs' complementary role in nutrition. Many herbs not only improve the flavor of food, but they also provide health advantages. For example, cinnamon has been demonstrated to boost insulin sensitivity, while bitter melon may help lower blood sugar levels.

Including these medicinal herbs in your diet can help manage diabetes and improve overall health.

Understanding diabetes and its care is a complicated journey that includes a variety of aspects, ranging from the disease's basic causes to the significance of lifestyle and diet. With an estimated 537 million adults living with diabetes globally, there is an urgent need for effective management techniques that enable people to take control of their health.

Conventional diabetes therapies, such as medications and lifestyle changes, lay the groundwork for successful management. However, the importance of nutrition cannot be emphasized; it is a necessary component that can significantly affect blood sugar levels and overall well-being. Individuals with diabetes can improve their health and quality of life by following dietary guidelines, appreciating the importance of food choices, and adding healing herbs.

Chapter 2: Herbal Remedies for Diabetes

As the search for alternative and complementary medicines gathers traction, herbal remedies are emerging as significant allies in the management and potential reversal of diabetes. This chapter discusses the most important factors for selecting herbs, followed by a summary of successful herbal treatments that have shown promise in managing blood sugar levels, enhancing insulin sensitivity, and promoting overall health.

Factors to Consider When Choosing Herbs for Diabetes

When it comes to choosing herbal medicines for diabetes, you need consider many crucial factors. The herbs' effectiveness, safety, and practicality are critical in ensuring that they benefit your health journey. Here are the key factors to consider:

Scientific Evidence and Research Support

Herbal selection should be based on scientific study and clinical data. Look for studies that show that herbs can help manage blood sugar levels, improve insulin sensitivity, and reduce problems linked with diabetes. Peer-reviewed journals, clinical trials, and respectable health organizations are all potential sources of research. The more compelling the research, the more certain you can be about the herb's potential advantages.

Traditional Use and Historical Context

Healing Herbs for Diabetes

Many plants have been utilized for ages in traditional medical systems, including Ayurveda, Traditional Chinese medical (TCM), and Native American healing techniques. Understanding the historical context and traditional applications of herbs might provide useful information about their medicinal potential. Herbs with a long history of use for diabetes treatment may contain mechanisms that are consistent with current scientific findings.

Safety and Side Effects

The safety profile of herbs is crucial. Investigate possible adverse effects, contraindications, and drug interactions. Some herbs may boost the effects of diabetic drugs, resulting in hypoglycemia (low blood sugar), whilst others may produce gastrointestinal distress or allergic responses. Before adding additional herbs to your regimen, consult with a healthcare expert, especially if you are currently using diabetes drugs.

Quality and Sourcing

The quality of herbal products might vary greatly. Choose herbs from recognized sources that follow good manufacturing procedures (GMP). Choose organic herbs wherever feasible, as they are less likely to contain pesticides or other dangerous chemicals. Consider whether you like whole herbs, tinctures, teas, or capsules, as this will influence your decision.

Personal Preferences and Lifestyle

Individual tastes and lifestyle considerations should also influence your choices. Some plants may have a strong taste or odor that might not appeal to everyone. Choose herbs that you enjoy eating and that fit well into your everyday routine. Whether you choose to make herbal teas, cook with fresh herbs, or take supplements, making sure they are compatible with your lifestyle can increase adherence and efficacy.

Consultation with healthcare providers

Before adopting herbal medicines into your diabetes management strategy, you should contact with a healthcare physician, preferably a licensed herbalist or registered dietitian who is familiar with herbal therapy. They can assist you in developing an approach that is tailored to your unique health needs and prescription regimen, ensuring that herbs are safely and effectively integrated into your lifestyle.

Overview of Effective Herbs: A Short Introduction to Key Herbs Used in Diabetes Management

With a better grasp of the selection criteria, let's look at some of the most beneficial herbs for diabetes treatment. Each of these herbs has been examined for its distinct qualities, which can aid in blood sugar regulation, insulin sensitivity, and other health advantages.

Cinnamon (Cinnamomum Verum)

Cinnamon is one of the most extensively examined herbs for diabetes treatment. According to several studies, cinnamon may increase insulin sensitivity and lower fasting blood glucose levels. Cinnamon's active components, including cinnamaldehyde, are thought to improve cellular glucose absorption and blood sugar regulation.

Healing Herbs for Diabetes

Adding cinnamon to your diet can be as simple as putting it on porridge, yogurt, or smoothies.

Bitter Melons (Momordica charantia)

Bitter melon has a long history of usage in traditional medicine to treat diabetes. It contains chemicals that act similarly to insulin, lowering blood sugar levels. Bitter melon has been demonstrated in studies to enhance glucose tolerance and lower blood sugar rises after meals. Bitter melon can be ingested as juice, prepared food, or a supplement.

Fenugreek (Trigonella foenum-graecum).

Fenugreek seeds contain soluble fiber, which may help control blood sugar levels by reducing carbohydrate absorption in the digestive tract. Studies have shown that fenugreek can considerably lower fasting blood glucose levels and improve glycemic management. You can add fenugreek into your diet by boiling the seeds or consuming them powdered.

Ginseng (panax ginseng)

Ginseng has been utilized for millennia due to its adaptogenic characteristics and general health benefits. According to research, ginseng may help enhance insulin sensitivity and lower blood glucose levels. Its revitalizing effects may also be good for people dealing with diabetes-related weariness. Ginseng is available in a variety of formats, including teas, extracts, and capsules.

Aloe Vera (Aloe Barbadensis Miller)

Aloe vera is well-known for its soothing characteristics, but it has also received attention for its possible impact on blood sugar regulation. Some studies have shown that aloe vera juice can considerably lower fasting blood glucose levels and enhance lipid profiles. Adding aloe vera to smoothies or drinking it as juice is a delightful way to get this herb into your diet.

Turmeric (Curcuma Longa)

The main ingredient in turmeric, curcumin, has anti-inflammatory and antioxidant characteristics that may assist diabetics. According to research, curcumin can improve insulin sensitivity while also lowering blood glucose levels. Turmeric can be easily added to curries and soups, or taken as a supplement, to get its health advantages.

Holy Basil (Ocimum Sanctum)

Holy basil, also known as Tulsi, is a beloved herb in Ayurvedic medicine due to its adaptogenic characteristics. Some research suggests that holy basil can help decrease blood sugar levels and enhance metabolic health. Holy basil can be enjoyed as a tea or used in cooking to offer flavor and health benefits.

Nopal cactus (Opuntia spp.

Nopal cactus, commonly called prickly pear, is high in fiber and antioxidants. Research suggests that it can help reduce blood sugar levels and enhance glycemic management. Nopal can be eaten fresh in salads, mixed in smoothies, or taken as a supplement.

Milk thistle (silybum marianum)

Milk thistle is well-known for its liver-supporting effects, but it also has potential in diabetes treatment. Silymarin, the active component of milk thistle, may help enhance insulin sensitivity and reduce blood sugar levels. It is available as a supplement, but you can also consume it as a tea or tincture.

Ginger (zingiber officinale)

Ginger is a popular cooking spice that contains anti-inflammatory and antioxidant qualities. Some research suggests that ginger may help lower fasting blood glucose levels and increase insulin sensitivity. Fresh ginger can be added to smoothies, stir-fries, or boiled into tea for a warming drink.

The potential for natural therapies in diabetes management is enormous and exciting. Individuals can improve their diabetes control techniques by understanding the criteria for selecting herbs and researching the many beneficial options available. These herbs not only have the potential to manage blood sugar levels, but they also give a variety of other health advantages that improve overall well-being.

As we progress through this book, we will delve further into cultivation techniques, practical applications, and recipes that will enable you to harness the healing power of herbs in your daily life. By adding these natural solutions into your daily routine, you can take proactive measures towards better health and potentially reverse the effects of diabetes.

Chapter 3: Key Healing Herbs.

In the continuous war against diabetes, nature has provided us with a treasure trove of healing herbs that have the capacity to manage and even reverse this chronic condition. This chapter digs into major medicinal herbs, explaining their health advantages, active ingredients, preparation methods, and use in daily life. With a focus on evidence-based insights and practical applications, you'll learn how these herbs can help you manage your diabetes.

1. Bitter Melons (Momordica charantia)

Health Benefits and Active Compounds

Bitter melon, often known as "bitter gourd," is a tropical fruit recognized for its peculiar flavor and several health advantages. Bitter melon includes various bioactive chemicals, including charantin, polypeptide-p, and vicine, which have been found in studies to imitate insulin and enhance glucose uptake in the cells. According to studies, regular use of bitter melon can result in considerable reductions in fasting blood sugar levels and an overall improvement in glycemic management. In addition, bitter melon has been linked to improved lipid profiles and increased antioxidant activity, which can aid diabetes patients reduce oxidative stress.

Preparation Techniques and Dosage Recommendations

Bitter melon can be ingested in a variety of ways, including fresh juice, cooked meals, and supplements. For individuals unfamiliar with its flavor, beginning with little doses, such as 100-200 grams of raw bitter melon per day, may be good. To make bitter melon juice, combine the fruit with water and drain it. Bitter melon juice is typically recommended to be consumed on an empty stomach for the best results. Cooked bitter melon can also be added to stir-fries or curries to get its advantages without the bitterness.

2. Fenugreek (Trigonella foenum-graecum).

Mechanism of Action and Use

Fenugreek seeds contain soluble fiber, which helps regulate blood sugar levels. The seeds include 4-hydroxyisoleucine, a chemical that has been demonstrated to increase insulin production and improve glucose tolerance. According to research, fenugreek can considerably lower fasting blood glucose and HbA1c levels in diabetics, making it an effective blood sugar management tool.

Recipes Including Fenugreek

Fenugreek can be a tasty and simple addition to your diet. One simple method to reap its benefits is to make fenugreek tea. To prepare, soak one teaspoon of fenugreek seeds in boiling water for 10-15 minutes. Strain the tea and add honey or lemon to taste. Fenugreek seeds can also be cooked into curries, soups, and stews. Another alternative is to crush the seeds and add them to smoothies or porridge for a nutritional boost.

3. Cinnamon (Cinnamomum Verum)

Anti-diabetic Properties and Studies

Cinnamon is a popular spice that not only adds flavor but also has numerous health advantages. Numerous studies have found that cinnamon can boost insulin sensitivity and reduce fasting blood glucose levels. Cinnamaldehyde, the active chemical, is thought to play an important role in

Healing Herbs for Diabetes

anti-diabetic actions via increasing glucose absorption and insulin signaling pathways.

Suggested Cinnamon Intake Strategies

Cinnamon is an easy and adaptable addition to your everyday routine. Ground cinnamon can be sprinkled on porridge, yogurt, or smoothies to enhance flavor and health benefits. Cinnamon can also be incorporated into herbal drinks or used to season savory dishes like stews and roasted vegetables. Some people choose to use cinnamon pills, but it is critical to contact with a healthcare expert before beginning any new supplement program.

4. Ginseng (panax ginseng)

Benefits of Blood Sugar Control

Ginseng has been used for therapeutic purposes for ages, particularly in Traditional Chinese Medicine. According to research, ginseng may help diabetics lower their blood sugar levels and enhance insulin sensitivity. Ginsenosides, the active components in ginseng, are thought to improve glucose metabolism and lower insulin resistance. Furthermore, ginseng may help alleviate diabetes-related exhaustion and boost overall energy levels.

Safety and interactions with other medications

While ginseng is generally considered safe, it should be noted that it may interact with medicines, particularly blood thinners and diabetes treatments. As a result, before introducing ginseng into your regimen, you must consult with a healthcare expert.

5. Aloe Vera (Aloe Barbadensis Miller)

Evidence of efficacy in diabetes management

Aloe vera is more than simply a popular cosmetic component; it has also received attention for its possible benefits in diabetes treatment. Research has revealed that aloe vera can considerably lower fasting blood glucose levels and improve glycemic management. The polysaccharides included in aloe vera, notably glucomannan, are thought to play an important role in its blood sugar-lowering properties.

How To Consume and Apply Aloe Vera

Aloe vera can be ingested in a variety of ways, including juice and gel. Look for juice that is 100% aloe vera and contains no additional sugars or artificial additives. A usual dose is 2-4 tablespoons per day. Furthermore, aloe vera gel can be administered topically to relieve skin irritations and promote healing. Ensure that you use high-quality items or extract fresh gel from the plant's leaves.

6. Gymnema Sylvestre.

Traditional Applications and Modern Research Findings

Gymnema sylvestre has a long history of usage in Ayurvedic medicine to treat diabetes. This plant's leaves are believed to lessen sugar cravings and blood sugar levels. Gymnema has been shown in studies to enhance glycemic control and perhaps repair insulin-producing cells in the pancreas.

How to Incorporate into Your Daily Routines

Healing Herbs for Diabetes

Gymnema sylvestre is widely available in supplement form, such as capsules and teas. Taking gymnema pills before meals may help people manage their sugar cravings. Additionally, gymnema tea can be made by steeping dried leaves in hot water. Incorporating gymnema into your regimen can help lower the need for sugary foods while also promoting overall blood sugar stability.

7. Turmeric (Curcuma Longa)

Active Ingredients and Benefits

Turmeric is known for its brilliant yellow color and potent chemical ingredient, curcumin. This herb is known for its anti-inflammatory and antioxidant capabilities, making it an important part of any diabetic care approach. Curcumin has been demonstrated to improve insulin sensitivity while lowering fasting blood glucose levels.

Culinary Uses and Supplements

Turmeric can add flavor to your diet while also being healthy. Turmeric can be used in curries, soups, and rice dishes, or it can be blended into smoothies to offer a pop of color. Curcumin capsules are commonly accessible for individuals who prefer supplements; nevertheless, it is recommended that formulations include black pepper extract (piperine) to improve absorption.

8. Holy Basil (Ocimum Sanctum)

Stress Relief Properties and Metabolic Effects

Holy basil, commonly known as Tulsi, is valued in Ayurvedic medicine for its adaptogenic characteristics, which aid the body in stress management. Stress can have a bad effect on blood sugar levels, hence holy basil is an important plant for diabetics. According to studies, holy basil may help reduce blood glucose levels and improve metabolic health.

How to Consume Holy Basil

Holy basil can be ingested in a variety of ways, including tea, pills, and fresh leaves. To make holy basil tea, simmer fresh or dried leaves in boiling water for 10 minutes before straining and enjoying. Incorporating fresh leaves into salads or smoothies is another tasty way to receive the benefits.

9. Milk thistle (silybum marianum)

Benefits of Liver Health and Diabetes

Milk thistle is best recognized for its liver-supportive characteristics, but new research reveals that it may also help people with diabetes. The chemical ingredient silymarin has been found to increase insulin sensitivity and lower blood sugar levels. Furthermore, milk thistle's antioxidant properties protect the liver from the harm caused by high blood sugar levels.

Preparation and Dosage Guidelines

Milk thistle comes in a variety of forms, including capsules, tinctures, and tea. The typical dosage for milk thistle extract is 140-420 mg of silymarin per day, divided into two to three doses. For those who like tea, steeping dried milk thistle seeds in hot water can produce a calming and healthy beverage.

Understanding the various medicinal herbs available for diabetes management is an important step toward gaining control of your health. Each

Healing Herbs for Diabetes

plant covered in this chapter has distinct qualities and benefits that can help regulate blood sugar and improve overall health. By including these herbs into your everyday routine, you can effectively supplement your diabetes control plan with natural elements.

As we continue to explore the world of herbal cures, the following chapter will include information on how to cultivate these healing plants, ensuring that you may get fresh, effective treatments right from your own garden. The journey to greater health through nature's bounty is only beginning!

Chapter 4: Growing Healing Herbs.

Growing your own medicinal herbs not only allows you to take responsibility of your health, but it also ties you to nature. An herbal garden can be a place of leisure, creativity, and wellness, as well as a source of fresh ingredients to supplement your daily life. In this chapter, we'll look at how to grow your own therapeutic herbs, with a focus on selecting the correct plants, preparing your soil, and ensuring the quality of your crop.

Starting Your Herbal Garden

Choosing the Right Herbs for Your Environment.

The first step in starting your herbal garden is deciding which herbs are best suited to your

Healing Herbs for Diabetes

environment. Consider the climate, available sunlight, and garden area. Here are a few suggestions to help you choose wisely:

Climate Compatibility: Learn about the herbs that flourish in your climate. For example, herbs like basil, oregano, and mint enjoy warm climates, whereas cilantro and parsley can endure cooler temps.

Sunlight Requirements: Most herbs require at least 6-8 hours of sunlight everyday. Herbs like rosemary and thyme flourish in direct sunlight, although others like chives and mint may tolerate partial shade.

Space Considerations: Determine whether you have enough space for a typical garden or if you'll need to use pots or containers. Many herbs thrive in pots, making them ideal for small balconies or patios.

Personal Preference: Think about the herbs you prefer cooking with or using for health advantages. Garlic, thyme, and peppermint are excellent starting herbs.

Basic Gardening Tips for Beginners

Starting your herbal garden doesn't have to be frightening. Here are some important gardening suggestions for beginners:

Start small: Choose a few herbs that you use frequently. As your confidence grows, you can expand your garden with different varieties.

Quality Seeds or Plants: Buy high-quality seeds or starting plants from a reliable nursery. Look for organic choices to ensure you're producing healthy, pesticide-free herbs.

Healing Herbs for Diabetes

Planting Depth: Refer to the planting directions for each herb. In general, seeds should be planted 2-3 times their diameter, while seedlings should be planted at the same depth as they were in their pots.

Herbs prefer continuous hydration, but not waterlogged soil. Water your herbs frequently, allowing the top inch of soil to dry between waterings.

Mulching: Adding a layer of organic mulch helps maintain soil moisture, suppresses weeds, and improves soil quality as it breaks down.

Soil Preparation and Care

Importance of Soil Quality and Organic Practice

Your herbal garden's success is heavily influenced by the quality of its soil. Healthy soil is nutrient-dense, well-drained, and has a thriving community of beneficial microbes. How to Prepare and Care for Your Soil:

Evaluating Soil Quality: Consider evaluating your soil's pH and nutrient levels. Most herbs like slightly acidic to neutral soil (pH 6.0 to 7.0). Soil test kits are available in garden centers and online.

Amending the Soil: Depending on the results, you may need to add organic matter, such as compost or well-rotted manure, to increase fertility and drainage. Incorporating organic matter can improve soil structure and moisture retention.

Using Organic Practices: Avoid using synthetic fertilizers and pesticides in your garden. Instead, use natural compost, cover crops, and organic pest management measures to keep the environment healthy.

Crop Rotation: If you plant herbs in the same location year after year, consider crop rotation.

This approach helps to prevent soil nitrogen depletion while also reducing insect and disease burden.

Harvesting and storing herbs

Best Practices to Maintain Potency

Harvesting your herbs at the right time and keeping them correctly is critical to preserving their flavor and potency. Here are some tips to make the most of your herbs:

Timing Your Harvest: The greatest time to harvest herbs is early in the morning, after the dew has evaporated but before the heat of the day sets in. This is when the essential oils are at their most concentrated. To encourage future growth in leafy herbs, snip off the top leaves.

Avoiding Overharvesting: When harvesting, take no more than one-third of the plant at a time. This ensures that the plant continues to develop and produce.

Fresh herbs can be stored in a jar of water as a bouquet, wrapped loosely with a plastic bag, and refrigerated. Alternatively, wrap them in a moist paper towel and store in a sealed plastic bag.

Drying Herbs: Drying is a great way to conserve herbs for a long time. To dry herbs, bundle them and hang them upside down in a cold, dark, and dry location. Once dried, keep them in sealed containers away from light to preserve their flavor and efficacy.

Freezing Herbs: Another alternative is to freeze herbs for future use. Chop your herbs, combine them with some water or olive oil, and pour into ice cube trays. Once frozen, place the cubes in a freezer bag for convenient use in cooking.

Healing Herbs for Diabetes

Cultivating your own therapeutic herbs is a satisfying undertaking that not only improves your culinary creations but also promotes your health and wellness. You may grow a successful herbal garden that provides fresh, effective medicines by selecting the perfect herbs for your climate, preparing high-quality soil, and using proper harvesting and storing practices.

Chapter 5: Using Herbs in Daily Life.

Incorporating therapeutic herbs into your daily routine can improve not only your diet, but also your general health. This chapter will look at many methods to use herbs, such as simple dishes that add taste and health benefits to your diet, as well as herbal drinks and medicines that provide natural diabetes management alternatives. Herbs' adaptability may transform your kitchen into a healing environment, with each recipe providing sustenance for both body and soul.

Incorporating herbs into meals

Simple Recipes using Healing Herbs

Herbs are culinary jewels that may enhance the flavor of any dish while also providing several

Healing Herbs for Diabetes

health advantages. Here are some easy recipes that emphasize the medicinal qualities of often used herbs:

Bitter Melon Stir-Fry

Bitter melon is known for its ability to reduce blood sugar levels. This stir-fry is quick and full of flavor.

Ingredients:

1 medium bittermelon, cut

2 tablespoons olive oil.

One onion, sliced

2 garlic cloves, minced

1 bell pepper, sliced

Add soy sauce to taste.

Add salt and pepper to taste.

Instructions:

In a medium-sized pan, heat the olive oil. Add the onion and garlic, and cook until aromatic.

Stir in the bitter melon and bell pepper, and cook for about 5 minutes, or until soft.

Season with soy sauce, salt, and pepper as desired. Serve heated with brown rice or quinoa.

This dish not only offers diversity to your meals, but it also contains bitter melon, which has several health benefits.

Fenugreek Seed Smoothie

Studies have indicated that fenugreek seeds can help manage diabetes and improve insulin sensitivity. Here's a wonderful smoothie to begin your day:

Healing Herbs for Diabetes

Ingredients:

1 tablespoon fenugreek seeds, steeped overnight.

1 banana.

1 cup almond milk (or milk of your choice)

One tablespoon honey (optional)

A pinch of cinnamon.

Instructions:

Drain and rinse the soaked fenugreek seeds.

Combine all ingredients and blend until smooth. Enjoy right away.

This smoothie not only tastes delicious, but it is also an effective method to get fenugreek into your diet.

Cinnamon-infused Quinoa Bowl

Cinnamon is known for its anti-diabetic qualities and can be simply incorporated to a variety of dishes. Try this warm quinoa bowl for breakfast.

Ingredients:

1 cup cooked quinoa.

1/2 cup almond milk.

1 teaspoon of cinnamon.

1 tablespoon of maple syrup (or honey).

Fresh fruits (such as berries and bananas)

Nuts or seeds for topping.

Instructions:

Healing Herbs for Diabetes

In a small pot, combine the cooked quinoa, almond milk, cinnamon, and sugar. Heat till warm.

Serve in a bowl, garnished with fresh fruits and nuts or seeds.

This breakfast bowl not only keeps you full but also helps you maintain stable blood sugar levels throughout the day.

Herbal Tea and Supplements

How to Prepare and Use Them Effectively.

Herbal drinks and pills make it easy to include herbs' medicinal powers into your everyday routine. Here are some suggestions for efficiently preparing and using herbal teas:

Bitter Melon Tea

To reap the benefits of bitter melon, prepare a calming tea:

Ingredients:

1 teaspoon of dried bittermelon leaves (or fresh slices)

1 cup boiled water

Instructions:

Place the bitter melon in a cup and cover with boiling water.

Steep for 5–10 minutes. Strain, and enjoy.

You can drink this tea every day to help control your blood sugar levels.

Fenugreek Tea

Healing Herbs for Diabetes

Fenugreek seeds can be used to make a nutritious tea.

Ingredients:

1 teaspoon of fenugreek seeds.

1 cup boiled water

Honey or lemon to taste (optional).

Instructions:

Crush the fenugreek seeds lightly to unleash their flavor.

Steep in boiling water for 10 to 15 minutes. Strain and sweeten as desired.

Drinking fenugreek tea on a regular basis helps improve digestion and metabolic health.

Cinnamon herbal infusion.

Cinnamon can also be infused to create a warm beverage.

Ingredients:

1 stick of Ceylon cinnamon (or one teaspoon ground cinnamon)

1 cup boiled water

Instructions:

Place the cinnamon stick in a cup and cover with boiling water.

Allow it to soak for 10 minutes before sipping.

Drinking this tea might deliver the advantages of cinnamon while keeping you warm.

Herbal Supplements.

Healing Herbs for Diabetes

If you prefer herbal supplements, look for high-quality extracts or capsules that contain the active ingredients of the herbs mentioned. Always consult with a healthcare practitioner before incorporating supplements into your regimen, especially if you are using drugs or have underlying health issues. Proper dose and timing are critical for maximizing benefits and limiting potential interactions.

Creating herbal remedies

Basic tinctures, extracts, and poultices

Making your own herbal remedies can be a powerful method to harness the healing abilities of plants. Here are some simple techniques to get started:

Herbal Tinctures

Tinctures are highly concentrated botanical extracts prepared from alcohol or vinegar. They are simple to produce and can be mixed into water or consumed immediately.

Ingredients:

One part dried herb (bitter melon, ginseng, or cinnamon).

5 parts high-proof alcohol (such as vodka or apple cider vinegar)

Instructions:

Place the dry herbs in a glass jar and fill with alcohol or vinegar.

Seal the jar tightly and store it in a cold, dark location for 4-6 weeks. Shake it occasionally.

Healing Herbs for Diabetes

Using a fine mesh strainer or cheesecloth, strain the liquid into a dark glass bottle. Store in a cool, dark area.

To reap the health benefits of the herbs, mix a few drops of tincture with water or consume it directly.

Herbal extracts

Herbal extracts are similar to tinctures, although they frequently contain glycerin or honey as a basis. These can be sweeter and simpler to eat.

Ingredients:

One part dried herb.

Three parts glycerin or honey.

Instructions:

In a container, combine the herb and the glycerin or honey.

Allow it to soak in a warm area for 4-6 weeks, shaking frequently.

Strain and place in a dark glass container.

This delicious extract can be added to teas, smoothies, or consumed directly for a delightful health boost.

Poultices

Poultices are externally applied to the skin and can relieve local discomfort or inflammation. Here's an easy method for making one:

Ingredients:

Fresh or dry herbs (ginger, aloe vera, or turmeric)

Water (enough to make paste)

Healing Herbs for Diabetes

Instructions:

Using a mortar and pestle or blender, grind the herbs into a paste, adding water as needed.

Apply the paste to the affected area and cover it with a clean towel.

Leave for 30-60 minutes before rinsing.

Poultices can provide localized relief and promote healing, particularly for skin problems or accidents.

Incorporating herbs into your daily routine is a joyful experience that provides both culinary enjoyment and health advantages. Whether you're cooking a delicious meal, sipping a calming herbal tea, or making your own cures, the choices are limitless.

As you continue to discover the realm of healing herbs, remember that patience and experimentation are essential. Embrace the process, listen to your body, and enjoy the natural benefits that herbs provide. In the following chapter, we will look at the larger aspects of holistic health, including how these practices can help you manage diabetes and improve your overall well-being. Your journey to maximum health via the power of herbs is only beginning!

Chapter 6: Lifestyle Changes for Diabetes Management.

Diabetes management extends beyond medication and natural therapies; it entails a comprehensive approach that includes nutrition, exercise, mindfulness, and regular blood sugar monitoring. In this chapter, we'll look at how to properly mix herbal medicines with healthy lifestyle choices to improve your diabetes management. We'll also talk about the importance of mental health and the best ways to check your blood sugar levels. By making these lifestyle adjustments, you can take proactive actions to protect your health and well-being.

Integrating Herbal Remedies, Diet, and Exercise

Developing a holistic approach

A holistic approach to diabetes treatment acknowledges the relationship between what you eat, how you move, and the herbs you incorporate into your daily routine. Integrating herbal medicines with a healthy diet and regular exercise will help you maintain stable blood sugar levels and general well-being.

Dietary choices

When choosing a diet for diabetes treatment, prioritize whole foods high in fiber, healthy fats, and lean proteins. Some diet regimens include:

Low glycemic index (GI) foods are absorbed more slowly, resulting in a gradual rise in blood sugar levels. Whole grains, legumes, non-starchy veggies, and most fruits are all good examples.

Healing Herbs for Diabetes

Incorporating Healing Herbs: As previously noted, herbs such as bitter melon, fenugreek, and cinnamon can be used to improve flavor and provide extra health benefits. For example, adding cinnamon to your daily porridge not only tastes good but also helps regulate blood sugar.

Balancing Macronutrients: Incorporate a variety of carbohydrates, proteins, and fats into each meal. This balance can help regulate blood sugar levels and increase satiety.

Exercise regimen

Physical activity is essential for controlling diabetes because it improves insulin sensitivity and aids in weight management. Here are some suggestions for incorporating fitness into your routine:

Aim for Regular Movement: Do at least 150 minutes of moderate aerobic activity per week, such as brisk walking, swimming, or cycling.

Incorporate Strength Training: Adding strength training activities two to three times per week can increase muscle mass and improve insulin sensitivity.

Consider Mind-Body Exercises: Yoga and tai chi can bring both physical and stress relief. These techniques also promote mindfulness, making them valuable additions to your diabetes treatment approach.

Herbal integrations

Incorporate Herbal Teas into Your Day: Begin your day with a cup of fenugreek tea or bitter melon tea to boost your metabolism and digestion.

Healing Herbs for Diabetes

Create Herbal-Infused Dishes: Use herbs not only for medical purposes, but also for their culinary diversity. Incorporate turmeric into smoothies, add fresh basil to salads, or make a stir-fry with ginseng and vegetables.

Combining these lifestyle factors results in a synergistic impact that improves blood sugar control. Tailoring your strategy to your unique tastes and demands will help you keep to your plan.

Mindfulness & Stress Management

The Effects of Mental Health on Diabetes

Diabetes management depends heavily on one's mental health. Stress can cause variations in blood sugar levels, making it critical to incorporate mindfulness activities into your daily routine.

Understanding Stress and Diabetes

When you are stressed, your body produces hormones like cortisol and adrenaline, which can raise blood sugar levels. Long-term stress can promote insulin resistance, making diabetes control more difficult. Recognizing the symptoms of stress and its effects on your health is the first step toward successful stress management.

Practicing mindfulness

Mindfulness activities can dramatically lower stress and improve emotional well-being. Here are a few strategies you can use:

Meditation: Set aside a few minutes each day to practice mindfulness meditation. Find a quiet place, close your eyes, and concentrate on your breathing. This technique might assist to relax your mind and lessen tension.

Deep breathing exercises can quickly reduce tension. Inhale deeply through your nose for four counts, then hold for four counts before exhaling through your mouth for four counts. Repeat many times to regain your center.

Gratitude Journaling: Keeping a gratitude diary allows you to reflect on the good things in your life. Writing down things you are grateful for every day will help you shift your focus away from difficulties and maintain a pleasant attitude.

Incorporating Yoga and Tai Chi

Yoga and tai chi are both effective stress-reduction and mindfulness exercises. These techniques blend moderate movements with breath control, which promotes relaxation and overall well-being.

Social Connections

Maintaining social relationships might also help reduce stress. Surround yourself with sympathetic friends and family who understand your situation. Consider attending a local diabetic support group to connect with people who are having similar issues.

You can improve your diabetes control by incorporating mindfulness and stress management strategies into your daily routine.

Monitoring Blood Sugar Levels.

Importance and Methods

Monitoring your blood sugar levels is an important part of diabetes care. Regularly monitoring your glucose levels allows you to learn how your body reacts to different diets, exercise, and lifestyle changes.

Understanding Blood Sugar Monitoring

Regular monitoring allows you to make more educated decisions about your food, exercise, and medications. It can also warn you about future issues, allowing you to take preventative measures to manage your health.

Selecting the Right Monitoring Method

Blood sugar levels can be monitored using a variety of methods, depending on your lifestyle and preferences:

Blood glucose meters: These devices provide immediate data and are widely used by diabetics. To use a meter, prick your finger to collect a drop of blood, which is then placed on a test strip and inserted into the meter.

Continuous Glucose Monitors (CGMs): These are wearable devices that constantly monitor your blood sugar levels throughout the day. They provide real-time data and can notify you of highs and lows, giving you a complete picture of your glucose trends.

A1C Testing: Your doctor may do an A1C test every three months to determine your average blood sugar levels over time. This test determines whether your diabetes treatment regimen is effective.

Establishing a Monitoring Routine

Make a blood sugar monitoring routine that suits your lifestyle. Here are some guidelines to maintain consistency:

Keep a record of your blood sugar readings, including the time of day and any relevant factors (for example, meals and activity). This information can help you detect patterns and make changes as needed.

Test at Key Times: It is critical to test before and after meals, before and after exercise, and whenever you experience symptoms. This exercise will provide you vital insights into how your body reacts to different triggers.

Communicate with Your Healthcare Team

During your doctor's appointments, share your blood sugar log with them. This information will allow them to adapt your treatment strategy and provide recommendations based on your specific needs.

Making lifestyle modifications is a powerful method to treat diabetes effectively. By combining herbal medicines with a healthy diet and regular exercise, you can construct a comprehensive approach to better health. Mindfulness and stress management are essential components that can improve your diabetes control by allowing you to face obstacles with confidence and clarity.

Finally, regular blood sugar monitoring will provide you with the information you need to make informed health decisions. As you embark on this journey to optimal well-being, keep in mind that every small change helps you live a better lifestyle. In the next chapters, we will look at the role of community support and continuous education in diabetes management, emphasizing the significance of being informed and engaged as you embark on your journey to health.

Chapter 7: Safety Considerations.

While herbal medicines can provide significant benefits for diabetes management, they should be used with caution. Understanding potential side effects, pharmaceutical interactions, and the necessity of individualized approaches can all contribute to safe and effective treatment. In this chapter, we will go over these key safety issues in detail, so you can make an informed decision about including herbs into your diabetes care plan.

Possible Side Effects of Herbs

Understanding Herb Safety

For millennia, herbs have been employed in traditional medical systems all across the world. However, they, like any other form of medication, can cause negative effects, particularly when taken incorrectly. Here are some common adverse effects to look for when utilizing herbal therapies.

Digestive Issues

Many plants have gastrointestinal effects. For example, bitter melon might produce stomach distress, diarrhea, or nausea in some people. Similarly, fenugreek may cause digestive discomfort, such as gas or bloating. Start with tiny doses and observe your body's reaction.

Allergic reactions.

Allergic responses can happen to any chemical, including plants. Rash, itching, and breathing problems are some of the possible symptoms. If you have a history of allergies, especially to plants or pollen, proceed with caution. When trying out a new topical herb, always perform a patch test first.

Healing Herbs for Diabetes

Hypoglycemia

Some plants, like ginseng and bitter melon, have strong blood sugar-lowering properties. While this can help manage diabetes, it can potentially cause hypoglycemia (low blood sugar) if not adequately controlled. The symptoms of hypoglycemia include dizziness, perspiration, confusion, and weakness. Regular blood sugar checks are necessary, especially when incorporating new herbs into your routine.

Hormonal Effects.

Certain herbs can have an effect on the body's hormone levels. Ginseng, for example, has been shown to influence estrogen levels, making it unsuitable for people who are hormonally sensitive. If you have any underlying hormonal concerns, you should contact with a doctor before taking these herbs.

Liver and Kidney Function.

Some herbs can have an impact on liver and kidney health, especially when used in large quantities. For example, large amounts of aloe vera might cause electrolyte imbalances and kidney problems. Always follow the recommended dosages and consult a doctor if you have any existing liver or kidney problems.

Monitoring Your Response

When incorporating any herbal therapy, it's critical to pay close attention to how your body reacts. Document any changes in your health, both favorable and negative, and communicate them with your healthcare physician. This proactive approach might help you discover potential side effects early on and change your regimen accordingly.

Interactions with medications

Importance of Consultation

Understanding the potential interactions between herbal medicines and prescribed pharmaceuticals is crucial to their safe use. Herbs can either enhance or reduce the effects of many medications, resulting in unforeseen consequences.

Understanding Herbal-Drug Interactions

Herbal remedies can alter how your body processes drugs. For example, St. John's Wort has been shown to interact with numerous antidepressants and blood thinners, potentially lowering their efficiency. Similarly, ginger can increase the effectiveness of anticoagulant drugs, raising the risk of bleeding.

Common Interactions:

Here are some possible interactions to be aware of:

Bitter Melon: This herb can drop blood sugar levels, which can cause hypoglycemia when taken with diabetic treatments such as insulin or sulfonylureas.

Fenugreek: Fenugreek can help decrease blood sugar and improve the effectiveness of diabetes treatments.

Cinnamon: High amounts of cinnamon can have an effect on liver enzymes, particularly when taken with drugs that are processed by the liver.

Healing Herbs for Diabetes

Ginseng: Ginseng can influence insulin levels and may interact with anticoagulant drugs.

Consulting Healthcare Providers

Always contact with your doctor before beginning any herbal cure, especially if you are taking prescription medications. Your healthcare professional can assist you in determining probable interactions and adjusting your treatment strategy accordingly. This teamwork is critical to ensuring safe and successful diabetes control.

Educate yourself.

It is critical to be knowledgeable about the herbs you intend to use. Investigate their potential interactions with the medications you are already taking. Many credible sources offer information on herb-drug interactions, allowing you to make informed judgments regarding your treatment options.

Personalized Approaches

Adapting Herbal Use to Individual Health Needs

Everyone's health is unique, so what works for one person may not work for another. Personalizing your approach to herbal treatments is essential for safe and efficient diabetes care.

Evaluating Individual Health Needs

When choosing herbs, think about your overall health, medical history, and specific diabetes treatment goals. For example, if you have a history of digestive disorders, you should avoid herbs that can aggravate the symptoms.

Starting Slow

When introducing new herbs, begin with small dosages and gradually increase as your body adapts. This method allows you to monitor your response while reducing the danger of negative effects. It's also a good idea to keep a journal of your experiences, recording any changes in blood sugar levels, side effects, or overall well-being.

Working with a qualified herbalist.

If you're not sure which herbs to take or how to safely incorporate them into your regimen, talk to a skilled herbalist or naturopath. These professionals can evaluate your health and design a herbal regimen to meet your specific requirements. They can also offer advice on doses and preparation techniques.

Incorporating lifestyle factors

Remember that herbs are only one component of a comprehensive diabetic control regimen. Diet, exercise, and stress management are all important lifestyle elements that influence overall health.

Collaborate with healthcare providers to develop a complete plan that incorporates herbal remedies into your daily routine.

Staying informed

Keep up to date on latest research and insights about herbal medicines and diabetes treatment. Staying informed will allow you to make better choices about your health and treatment alternatives.

Incorporating herbal treatments into your diabetes treatment strategy can be an effective tool for improving your health. However, safety must always be a priority. Understanding potential side effects, recognizing combinations with drugs, and adapting your strategy to particular health needs allow you to get the benefits of herbal therapies while reducing dangers.

Healing Herbs for Diabetes

Maintain a proactive approach to your health journey. Engage with healthcare practitioners, be informed, and listen to your body's cues. In the next chapters, we will look at the role of community support and continual education in diabetes care, highlighting the benefits of connection and shared knowledge as you journey toward wellness.

Conclusion

Empowerment via Knowledge

As we come to the end of our tour through the realm of herbal remedies for diabetes management, it's important to consider the power that knowledge brings. Throughout this book, we've looked at the complex relationship between herbs and health, revealing the power of natural therapies to supplement conventional treatments and improve overall well-being. This exploration is about more than just learning certain plants or cures; it's about giving yourself the tools you need to make informed health decisions.

Knowledge is the first step towards empowerment. The more you understand about

Healing Herbs for Diabetes

herbs that can help manage diabetes, the more confident you will be in making decisions that are in line with your health objectives. Understanding how these herbs operate might change the way you approach diabetes management, whether you're blending bitter melon into your morning smoothie or making a calming cup of cinnamon tea.

Furthermore, this understanding enables you to advocate for yourself during talks with healthcare providers. Understanding the potential benefits and limitations of herbal medicines enables you to have meaningful talks about your treatment options, ensuring that you play an active role in your health journey. Remember that your body is your finest teacher; follow your instincts and be curious about how different cures effect your health.

Last Thoughts on Managing Diabetes Naturally

This book has covered a variety of topics related to healthily controlling diabetes, with an emphasis on a holistic approach that incorporates nutrition, exercise, and herbal therapies. Here are some crucial lessons to consider as you begin your journey:

Holistic Approach: Diabetes management is not a one-size-fits-all solution. It involves a diverse strategy that includes food, physical activity, stress management, and natural medicines. Each element is essential for maintaining stable blood sugar levels and overall health.

Using Herbs Wisely: While herbs can provide substantial benefits, they should be used with prudence. Understand the potential side effects

Healing Herbs for Diabetes

and interactions with drugs, and always talk with a doctor before incorporating new herbs into your routine. This proactive approach guarantees that you make safe choices based on your specific health needs.

Nutrition is important: A well-balanced diet is essential for managing diabetes. Eating complete, nutrient-dense foods and limiting processed sweets can dramatically enhance your health. Herbs like fenugreek and cinnamon not only provide flavor but also help with blood sugar regulation, making them ideal complements to your diet.

Stay Engaged and Informed: The field of herbal medicine is always evolving. Stay involved by researching new discoveries, attending workshops, or joining local herbalist communities. The more you know, the more prepared you will be to make informed decisions that benefit your health.

Self-Care is Critical: Don't overlook the role of self-care in your diabetes treatment strategy. Prioritize mindfulness, stress alleviation, and mental well-being because they can all have a big impact on your overall health and blood sugar levels. Regular physical activity, such as yoga or meditation, might help you relax and balance out your herbal routine.

Community Support: Do not underestimate the importance of community. Surround yourself with supportive friends, family, or groups that understand your situation. Sharing your experiences, insights, and triumphs with others can encourage and motivate you to continue working toward your health objectives.

To summarize, naturally controlling diabetes is a pleasant journey full of opportunity for personal growth and discovery. Embrace the power of knowledge, investigate herbal cures with curiosity, and take a proactive attitude to health.

Healing Herbs for Diabetes

Every step you take to better understand your body and its requirements is a step toward empowerment.

Remember, you are not alone on this journey. Many others have had similar experiences and struggles, and together, you may form a supportive network that promotes recovery and wellness. By delving into the world of herbal treatments, you are opening yourself up to a plethora of possibilities that can improve your quality of life.

Allow this conclusion to act as an invitation to continue your educational and self-improvement journey. The ability to control diabetes naturally is within you, and with the correct education, tools, and support, you can thrive on your health journey. Embrace the journey, be curious, and remember that every minor change helps your general well-being. Here's to your health and the empowering journey that lies ahead!

J. Waller

The end

Healing Herbs for Diabetes

www.ingramcontent.com/pod-product-compliance
Lightning Source LLC
Chambersburg PA
CBHW070155230526
45471CB00002B/670